Arthritis

Live With Less Pain and Inflammation

Tips and Techniques You Can Use to Lessen the Pain and Inflammation of Arthritis

RON KNESS

Contents

Introduction

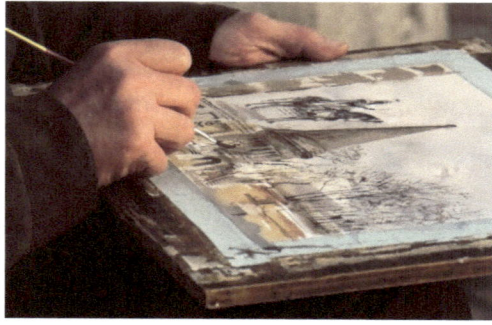

In this book, you will learn valuable information that will help you manage the pain and inflammation that comes along with arthritis, so that you can live an active, full life without debilitating pain.

In this first chapter, we are going to talk a little bit about the two most common types of arthritis, their symptoms and the best options for alleviating the pain and inflammation that they cause.

If you (as I do) or someone you know suffers from arthritis then I'm sure you're aware that it is a common disease that causes pain and inflammation. Severe cases have the power to rob sufferers of their freedom of mobility. There are many different types of arthritis and only a doctor can tell you which one you have. Most arthritis sufferers typically fall into one of two categories.

– Osteoarthritis

This is the one that I have and it is predominantly found in men and women over the age of 65, is also known as degenerative arthritis. This name comes from the progression of the disease. It beings with cartilage breakdown. The cartilage covering the bones degenerates and gradually wears away. Sufferers are left with exposed bones that rub against each other, causing severe pain and discomfort as well as difficultly of moving for many.

The most noticeable symptoms of osteoarthritis are joint pain, inflammation and stiffness which is common the morning and after physical activity. All joints can be impacted by osteoarthritis, but the most common are the hips, feet, back, knees, and fingers. Those with arthritis problems in the hands and feet may find it difficult to walk without a limp and grasp items that are otherwise easy to pick up.

As with most types of arthritis, there is not just one cause for osteoarthritis. There are many contributing factors. These include body weight, previous injuries, and genes. Although osteoarthritis typically affects the elderly, athletes who repeatedly use the same joints and suffer injury are at an increased risk.

As for body weight, the joints and muscle surrounding them carry most of the body's weight; more weight applies more pressure. Although rare, there are defects that can lead to osteoarthritis.

These include a lack of protein that makes up cartilage and the poor fitting of bones and joints.

– Rheumatoid Arthritis

The second type is rheumatoid arthritis affects over one million people in the United States. It doesn't discriminate, it effects people of all ages. In fact, there are three types of rheumatoid arthritis for juveniles alone. The cause? The immune system is supposed to protect our body, but in some cases, it does the exact opposite. With rheumatoid arthritis, it attacks the joint lining membrane.

The most noticeable symptom of rheumatoid arthritis is pain. If untreated, other complications can arise. The most common is disability. To prevent this from happening, all patients are urged to exercise their joints and muscles, even though it may be painful at first.

Another common symptom of rheumatoid arthritis is inflammation. The swelling can be mild to severe. In most instances, this is what separates rheumatoid arthritis from other forms. Swelling and inflammation is likely, but it is much more prominent and debilitating.

Most rheumatoid arthritis suffers rarely experience constant pain. The disease flares up from time to time. These flare ups are trigged by joint overuse and certain foods. As for the cause, it is currently unknown. There are however many theories. One being genes.

Now that you are familiar with the most common types of arthritis, what comes next? If you or someone who you know suffers from arthritis, medical care is essential. A proper diagnosis is important to developing the best treatment option. Low impact exercise can loosen the joints and strengthen the surrounding muscles.

This will help eliminate some of the joint stiffness, it can also prevent disability and deformities in chronic suffers.

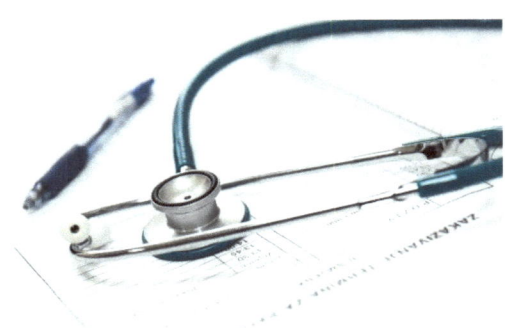

Some pain can be treated, but it will reoccur. Here are a few tips that can help you learn how to manage pain:

- Start by eliminating stress

- Ask for help when you need it

- Get plenty of sleep, and

- Learn how to relax.

While these are only general tips that sound almost too simple, they really can help.

Alleviating arthritis pain and inflammation is not an exact science. What works for one person may not work for another, so it is important to take care of your overall health in order help minimize its painful side effects.

One natural treatment that works for some people is the Paddison Program. You can read more about the program to see if it is for you at:

http://www.rheumatoidarthritisprogram.com/?hop=photo57.

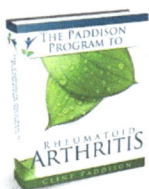

Over the Counter Medications and Products – Which Ones Really Work?

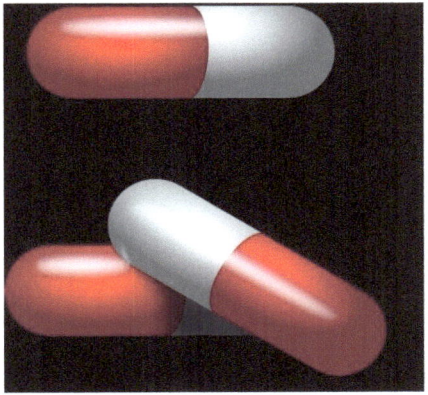

In the last chapter, we talked about two of the common types of arthritis and their treatment options. In this chapter, we are going to go over some of the pros and cons of over-the-counter arthritis medications.

When it comes to arthritis pain and discomfort, many patients want relief and they want it now. For many, the pain is unbearable and they are willing to try just about any over-the-counter product or natural remedy they can get their hands on, but are they your best option?

Arthritis pain relief comes in many different forms. Many turn to pain pills like Tylenol, Advil, Aleve, Bayer, or their generic counterparts. Then there are arthritis creams. These creams usually contain the active ingredient capsaicin.

You can find out more about capsaicin here:
http://www.webmd.com/drugs/2/drug-4181/capsaicin-top/details

Lastly, there are heating pads and patches. Heat has long been known to reduce the pain and discomfort associated with arthritis. For at-home care, a microwavable or electric heating pad works great. For on the go or in the car, onetime-use heating patches are very convenient.

Over-the-counter products are easy to purchase without a prescription and they are available just about anywhere. Heating pads, arthritis creams, and pain medications are available for sale both online and locally. In terms of local shopping, your options include health food stores, department stores, drug stores, and supermarkets.

Most over-the-counter products provide quick relief. With the exception of Tylenol Arthritis, which is designed to provide both fast and long-lasting pain relief, it can take up to fifteen minutes for the medicine to kick in. When in pain, this may seem like a lifetime, but it is actually very quick. For the quickest relief, opt for arthritis creams. Many report pain relief as soon as the cream touches their skin!

While there are many good reasons why someone may opt for over-the-counter products, there are some downsides as well.

For instance, their costs can add up overtime. The more you use a product, the more you need to buy. In terms of pain reliever, look for large packages, as they tend to cost less. If possible, buy in bulk. As for the heating patches and pouches, the patches are ideal for on-the-go travel, but don't use them at home. Instead, opt for a heating pad that you can continue to reuse. In the end, you get a better value for your money.

You can also help lower the cost of over-the-counter products by shopping at discount retailers and clubs like Sam's and Costco. Coupons and sales can also lessen the costs.

Just keep in mind that while many over-the-counter products provide fast acting arthritis pain relief, it is often a short-term fix. This is nice, but remember that relief will not be long-lived. As soon as your medication wears off or when your heating pad loses heat, your pain will start to return.

For the ultimate long-term relief of arthritis pain, swelling, and stiffness, do more than just rely on over-the-counter products. Make sure you visit your physician for a proper diagnosis and they can often prescribe medication that when taken overtime will provide long-lasting relief. If these prove successful for your body, you may not need over-the-counter products daily - only when pain flares up.

Pain Management

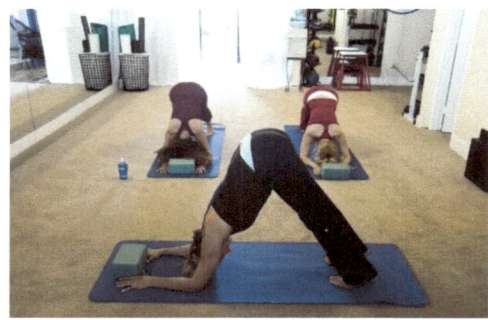

Anyone who suffers with arthritis knows pain management is important. Without it, you may be unable to function from day-to-day. Unfortunately, many home remedies and over-the-counter medications require money.

Although there are, many products available and you can purchase a bottle of pain medication for a few dollars, that may be money you just don't have to spare, and with long term use, the cost can add up fast. So, what should you do, just live with the pain? No, there are many ways to seek arthritis pain relief and many are free!

- Regular exercise

Right about now you may be thinking exercise isn't possible. After all, your joints are in pain. However, the majority of physicians recommend regular exercise for arthritis relief. Yes, this is true. Exercise can help and should be incorporated it your daily routine, not just those suffering from arthritis.

When it comes to arthritis, exercise does wonders for the body. It assists with weight loss and promotes healthy freedom of movement. This movement strengthens the muscles surrounding the joints, which provides extra protection and reinforcement.

One such method of exercise that works particularly well is yoga. Because it focuses on gentle movement that increase flexibility, it can bring some relief from the pain of arthritis

While exercise is necessary, it isn't always free. If you're on a budget, wisely plan your workouts. Instead of opting for a gym

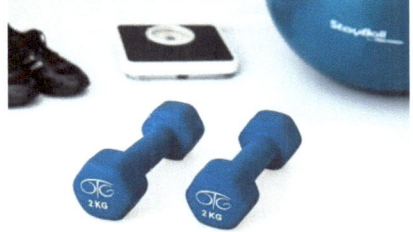 membership so you can use the treadmill, walk around your neighborhood or inside a shopping center. There are also excellent walking videos that you

can use in the comfort of your own home, like Walk Away the Pounds and don't forget to search YouTube for free Power Walk options.

Here is a website dedicated to walking from home: http://www.walkathome.com/

Instead of signing up for an aerobics class, turn on some music in your home and move around. Something as simple as stretching your fingers daily can provide long-term pain relief.

Although this exercise may be painful at first, it will get easier overtime. Remember any type of movement will reduce joint stiffness. This should not only provide pain relief, but it lessens the risk of additional complications. For individuals with arthritis who don't learn the benefit of the little or no treatment, they will later find themselves dealing with severe stiffness, the inability to move, and deformities. Combine diet and exercise to lose weight.

Right about now, you may be thinking dieting isn't free either. In reality it is. You already buy food and drinks. You need these to survive. Carefully choose your foods. Eliminate those high in fat and calories.

- **Weight loss**

Weight loss is an easy way to lessen the pain associated with

arthritis. The less weight you have pressing on the joints, the less pain you will experience. If you don't have any weight to lose that's good, but you still need to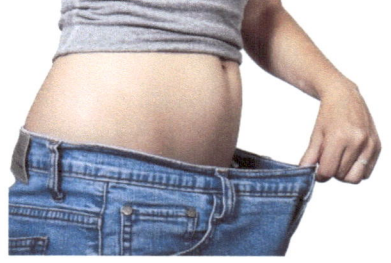

be aware of the importance and many health benefits of healthy eating.

Avoid applying too much pressure to the painful joints. Many suffering from severe arthritis will experience pain no matter what the activity, while others will only experience pain when triggered.

For example, individuals who have pain in their elbows should still exercise moderately but avoid lifting heavy items that can trigger a flair-up. They should also be careful to lift items properly.

Yes, it is easier to reach down and grab a box, but this can put undo strain the elbows. Instead, properly squat down and lift with your entire body. Avoiding joint pressure will not eliminate arthritis pain, but it will lessen the severity.

- Ask for help

As we have discusses before, some arthritis sufferers trigger severe pain by trying to complete tasks they shouldn't. If you have severe arthritis in your hands, don't spend hours trying to open a jar. Not only will you get frustrated with your inability to open it, you increase the risk of severe pain. Instead, ask for help.

Getting relief from arthritis symptoms doesn't have to be complicated or expensive. Just make sure you try to exercise regularly, eat healthy, limit strenuous activity, and ask for help. Doing so will lessen the pain you experience, without costing you a penny.

Tips to Help Control Arthritis

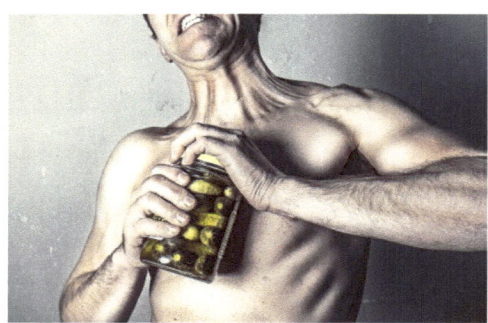

If you suffer from arthritis, you may not only experience joint pain and swelling, but difficulty functioning from day-to-day. Whether you are prone to occasional pain or experience it all the time, going about a normal day may seem like an impossible task, but it doesn't have to be.

Here are some thing you can do to make life a little easier:

First, make it easy to get around your home. If you suffer from arthritis of the toes, feet, hips, or knees, it's difficult to move. Walking from one room in your home to the next, may trigger pain so it's important to make it as easy as possible to navigate. If you have limited mobility, enlist the help of a trusted friend, family member, or neighbor to rearrange your furniture and create a straight path to the most used areas of your home. The less steps and turns you have to make, the better.

Regardless of which joints hurt, it can be difficult to reach and grip so make sure all the items you use the most are within easy reach. For instance, if you find it too difficult to reach to the top shelf in your kitchen cupboard place all foods and dishes on lower shelves and even if you have to utilize your countertops for convenience. By making your life at home easier, you will be able to manage and even prevent the discomfort and painful flare-ups associated with arthritis.

Keep pain relievers handy. As we discussed in a previous chapter, they typically provide relief in as little as 15 minutes. Some over-the-counter arthritis creams provide pain relief as soon as it meets the skin. Since they do work, keep them on hand. Keep some pills and creams in your home, car, and purse. There are many ways to reduce the risk of arthritis pain, but there are no guarantees. Anything can trigger a flair-up, so always be prepared.

If you suffer from arthritis of the toes, feet, hips, or knees, walking can be difficult and painful. With each step you take, pressure is applied to your already painful joints. You can lessen the pressure with walking aids. These may include knee braces, crutches, or canes. Remember, the less pressure you apply to your joints, the less pain you should feel.

Arthritis patients often experience times when they feel helpless. This is occurs over some of the simplest tasks that many people take for granted like not being able to open a jar of spaghetti sauce or walk to the mailbox without experiencing pain. It's very frustrating to be unable to handle daily tasks without pain. Although it can be hard, don't be afraid to ask for help. Ask your neighbor to deliver your mail to your home and save a heavy box until a family member can help you.

One of the many problems arthritis patients face is difficulty managing their pain. Talking about those difficulties can help. For most, the worst thing to do is to keep these emotions bottled up in side. It is best to talk to someone at home or join an arthritis support group. If you opt not to, keep a journal instead. Write down or record all feelings, including the good and the bad.

In short, there are many ways to treat and manage arthritis pain. Over-the-counter products are a lifesaver for many arthritis patients, but they are not your only option. The first step should be focusing on day-to-day tasks. When these seem easier and less painful, the rest will simply just fall into place.

Choosing the Right Supplements to Control Pain

If you suffer from arthritis, chances are you look high and low for

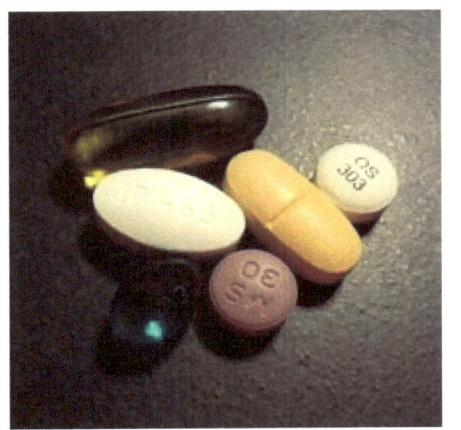

relief. It can be a constant struggle of trial and error trying to find an effective treatment. Did you know that certain herbal, dietary, and natural supplements could help relieve arthritis pain and discomfort?

Some not only reduce pain and discomfort, but swelling too. If this is new to you, you may want to run out and purchase a bottle of supplements, but wait! If this is your first time buying these supplements, you must first know some important things.

Not all supplements aid in arthritis relief. There are wide ranges of dietary, herbal, and natural supplements available for sale, both locally and online. Make sure you do your research first to determine what supplements may reduce your joint pain and swelling.

For instance, Avocado Soybean Unsaponifiables (ASU) is believed to slow down the making of inflammation causing chemicals. Devil's Claw can reduce inflammation and pain in arthritis patients. These are just a sample of the supplements that can help. Before heading to the health store, know what to buy.

When researching supplements or when browsing at the store, read

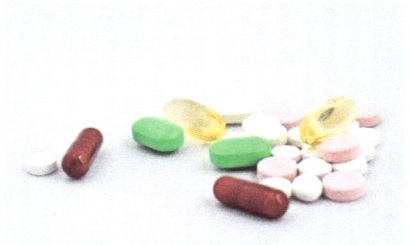 all packages. Most will outright state what the product can do. For example, capsules of Devil's Claw may state they assist with the reduction of arthritis pain and

swelling.

While arthritis has no permanent cure, you can learn to manage and temporarily treat the joint pain, stiffness, and swelling associated with it. When shopping for supplements be sure to avoid any product that claims it will cure your arthritis. This is an outright lie and usually a waste of money.

Herbal, natural, and dietary supplements are not like over-the-counter pain relievers. They rarely provide you with immediate relief. To see results they must be taken consistently overtime. Most reduce the likelihood of pain and inflammation, especially with regular and continued use.

Unfortunately, this means you may have to purchase and try many supplements. To prevent the costs from becoming too high, price compare. Find a quality, yet economical brand. Buy your supplements on sale, buy in bulk, use coupons, or shop at a store with good prices. Always compare price with quantity. A larger package of supplement capsules will cost more money, but it is usually a better value for that money.

- Doctor recommendations

Most arthritis patients fear discussing supplements with their physician. Most believe they will only hear discouragement. Not all physicians believe in or recommend the use of supplements, but don't be afraid to discuss this with your doctor. Many now embrace supplements, when used with prescribed or recommended medicine. So, tell your doctor you want to try ASU to reduce your joint swelling, but that you will continue to take your over-the-counter pain relievers for pain, as directed and see what s/he says.

- Drug interactions

Why is it important to speak with your physician about supplements? Some can interact with common medications. For example, the Devil's Claw mentioned above can counteract with diabetes medication, acid reducers, and blood thinners. Ask your doctor if the supplement you intend to take is risky with your current medications.

- Side effects

Most supplements come directly from nature, but not all things in nature are safe for all. Some supplements can have side effects. For instance, Gingko can reduce disease flare-ups for some. However, it does have many side effects. These include headaches, upset stomachs, and dizziness. Always be sure to look at the side effects for your preferred supplement before you begin taking them.

Many natural supplements can provide you with arthritis relief. Nevertheless, don't run out and buy the first supplement you see at the health store. Opt for a supplement that will not interact with your current medications, one that is affordable, one that has little to no side effects, and one that will treat your troubling arthritis symptoms.

Pain Relief Options for Osteoarthritis In the Knees

In the last chapter, we talked about how to choose the right supplement. In this one, we are going to go over some pain relief options for osteoarthritis in the knees.

If you are one of the millions of people who suffers from

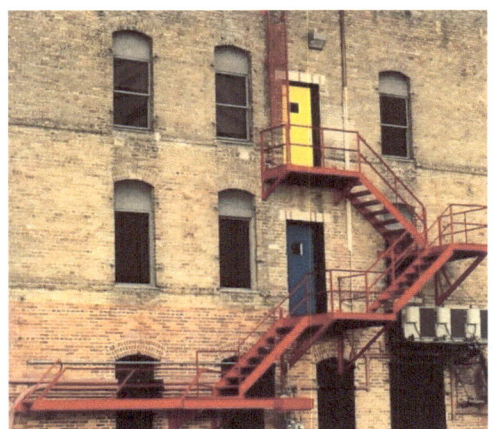

osteoarthritis in the knees then you know how painful it can be. Fortunately, your suffering doesn't have to be a constant reminder of how hard it can to simply walk across the room.

For osteoarthritis, most health care professionals recommend Acetaminophen (Tylenol). With that said, there are many over-the-counter pain relievers available. Choose a brand that you can afford and one that provides you with relief. For instance, if Naproxen (Aleve) or Ibuprofen (Motrin) works well for you, use it.

*Just, remember these types of medications are only meant for short-term relief, not long-term use. Be sure to follow the dosage instructions and read the warning information before usage. I finally had to go off of Aleve because it was starting to cause stomach ulcers.

Now I primarily manage my arthritis joint pain by using my hot tub set at 102 degrees for 20 minutes per day. It works for me and I'm not ingesting a bunch of medications.

Topical arthritis creams are also a good option for temporary relief. You simply apply the cream directly to the hurtful joints and it begins to work on contact. At first, you may notice a slight tingle or sting, but then comes the relief. This relief usually lasts as long as over-the-counter pain relievers.

As we have discussed before, when examining the active ingredients in over-the-counter arthritis creams, you are likely to find they contain capsaicin. This ingredient is also found in cayenne pepper. Many not only recommend a capsaicin cream, but adding the pepper spice to foods for flavor and additional health benefits.

Most physicians will only write prescriptions for severe pain. This pain cannot be treated with over-the-counter medications. Opioids like Tramadol and Oxycodone are two of the most common prescribed pain relievers, but keep in mind that they do come with a higher list of side effects as well as a risk of addiction or problems from improper use.

NOTE: Always, be sure to follow your doctor's advice when taking these types of medications. If you experience any side effect, contact them immediately.

– Heat

For most, heat provides pain relief. Draw a warm bath, use a warm washcloth, or purchase a heating pad. As always, caution is advised to prevent burns. Although most individuals benefit from heat, some do better with cold. Some medical professionals, according to Arthritis Today, recommended alternating between the two.

To reduce joint pain, strong muscle strength is needed. With strong muscles, you are able to rely on them and use them more. This puts less pressure on achy knees. In fact, strong muscles give the joints extra protection and cushion. Therefore, exercise is advised. If it is painful to exercise, start out slow with low-impact exercises.

For some, stretching and light walking is enough. If still too painful, consider low-impact water exercises.

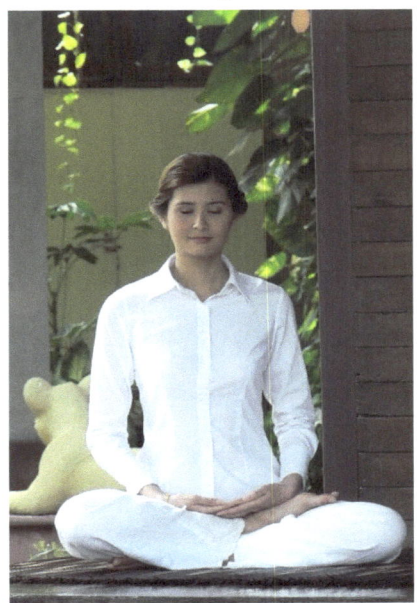

Some osteoarthritis patients may find it too painful to exercise. Your goal is to avoid and prevent pain, so why do something that causes it? Exercise has long-term health benefits.

Not only does it promote an overall healthy body, but also it provides the joints protection through increased muscle strength. You can exercise at home, but physical therapy is good. In some cases, this gives you easy access to water exercises. You can also learn safe low-impact exercises to do at home.

Not all patients suffering from osteoarthritis are overweight, but those who are increase the risk of pain. The more weight you carry around, the more pressure there is applied to the knees. As a matter-of-fact every extra 10 pounds of body weight puts an additional 30 pounds of pressure on the knees.

If you can lose weight without compromising your health, do so. The best way to lose weight is to combine exercise with healthy eating.

People who suffer from osteoarthritis in the knees are more likely to experience walking troubles. It can be painful to walk from one room to another, let alone leave the house. A knee brace can provide support and stability. A proper fitting knee brace not only makes it easier to walk, but less painful too! Knee braces are available for sale at most health and drugstores, but talk to your physician first.

Many arthritis patients believe they reach the point of no return. This is when the pain is so unbearable it seem as if nothing will work. Those individuals are more likely to suffer in silence than seek treatment.

If you are one of those individuals or if you just need a push to lose weight or exercise, a strong support system is vital. For many, talking about their pain helps to ease it. Ensure you have someone at home to discuss your arthritis with or find local support groups.

In the next chapter, we'll talk about how to determine whether surgery is an option for relieving arthritis pain or not.

Is Surgery Right for You?

If you have been recently diagnosed with arthritis or if you suspect

you have it, thoughts of surgery may automatically pop into your head. Yes, some patients must undergo surgery, but it is actually very rare. Despite the common belief, it is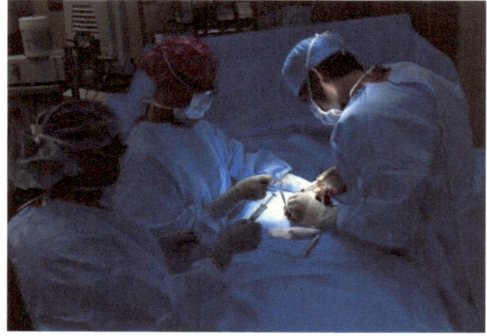

possible to treat and manage the symptoms of arthritis, such as joint pain, swelling, and difficulty moving, without surgery.

When is surgery an option?

- Unbearable Pain.

When the pain is so severe that over-the-counter pain relievers and prescription pain relievers don't work, surgery may be the last resort. Overtime, our bodies get use to the pain relievers we ingest. Overtime the Tylenol that once provided with you with relief may no longer do so. When that point arrives, speak to your doctor about prescribed medications. He or she will likely want to try those first before opting for surgery.

- Joint damage.

The elderly and those who let their arthritis go untreated, are susceptible to joint damage. This includes deformities. For example, a patient with severe rheumatoid arthritis may have bent fingers. This not only looks different, but it is excruciating in terms of pain. Surgery can be used to correct these deformities and other severe joint damage.

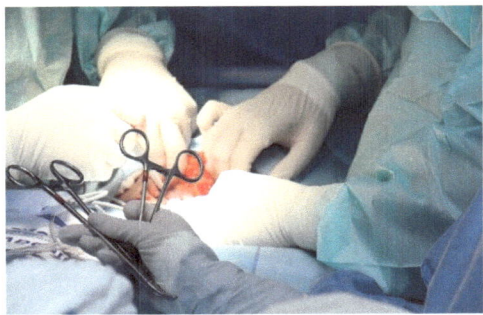

Now let's briefly go over some of the types of procedures available:

- Arthroscopy

This is a minimally invasive surgery and a great alternative to open surgery. A small incision is made in the skin. Then, a thin viewing instrument, known as an arthroscope is inserted towards the painful joint. Many surgeons use this procedure to diagnose a problem and decide on a course of treatment. It can also be used to perform small surgeries.

It has many benefits, including less pain, lower costs, and less hospitalization. So, if you need surgery, ask your doctor about arthroscopy as a suggestion.

- Arthrodesis

This surgery is very rare, as there is a high risk of complications. Moreover, it results in a permanent disability. So, why is it even offered? It is the only hope of pain relief for some individuals. These individuals have a diseased joint that cannot be fixed any other way. Pain and swelling are common and unmanageable. Arthrodesis involves fusing two bones into a joint. This prevents joint movement. For many, this is a last and only resort.

- Joint replacement

Joint replacement surgeries are common with the shoulders, knees, and hips. With joint replacement surgeries, the ends of nearby bones are replaced. This results in new joint surfaces. It will take time and physical therapy, but most patients experience a reduction and pain and an increase in mobility. For the fingers and toes, joint replacement is less common. Typically, surgeons opt for the fusion of smaller joints, as opposed to total replacement.

What are the alternatives to arthritis related surgery?

For starters, how severe is your arthritis? When were you diagnosed?

The earlier osteoarthritis and rheumatoid arthritis are diagnosed, the easier it is to treat without surgery. As we have discussed before, exercise is vital. Yes, it can be difficult to move your joints, so exercise may seem like it is out of the question, but it is very important to incorporate some type of physical activity into your daily routine.

Start with low impact exercises or opt for water exercises or physical therapy. The more a joint is moved, the less stiffness you will experience. This can also help reduce the chance of deformities.

As for the pain, remember that surgery is only used as a last resort. First, try over-the-counter pain pills and cream or ask for stronger prescription medications. Heat also helps many. Soak in a warm bath daily or use a heating pad. Although there is little scientific proof to back these claims, many arthritis patients report long-term relief with continued use of natural remedies and supplements, including cayenne pepper, pineapples, ASU, and ginger.

Do Topical Creams Work for Pain Relief?

As we well know, there are over one hundred different types of arthritis. Despite the different causes and symptoms they all have,

one thing is common and that is pain. All arthritis patients suffer pain in varying degrees. For some, it comes and goes. For others it's constant. You want relief and you want it 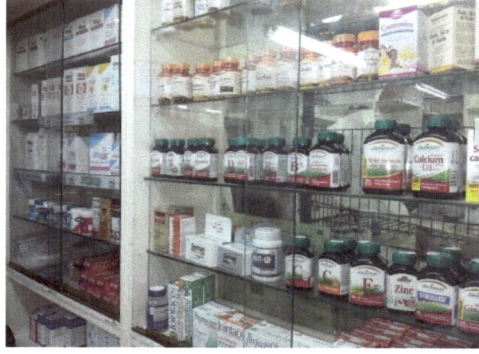 now, but is instant arthritis pain relief possible? The answer is, yes and no.

Before focusing on a few ways that you can get quick arthritis pain relief, it is important to note variances. It all depends on your definition of instant. For most, instant means right away and immediately, because when you are in pain, 15 minutes can literally feel like a lifetime. For others, 10 to 15 minutes is soon enough.

As we discussed in a previous chapter, in terms of over-the-counter arthritis relief, you have two main options:

- Over-the-counter pain pills

- Over-the-counter topical arthritis creams.

So, which provides you with the fastest relief? It all depends on your body.

Most pain relief capsules or tablets have to dissolve in your body to start working. It can take time for the entire pill to dissolve, which means they take a little longer to be effective. On the other hand, Advil has a Liquid-Gel capsules where just the outer layer needs to dissolve, so relief is typically faster. Tylenol has a special arthritis formula that has two dissolving layers; one is fast for quick relief and the second is slower for long-lasting relief.

When it comes to topical creams, most see relief right away. In fact, you may experience relief as soon as the cream makes contact with the skin. Even if you have never used these creams before, you may have used Bengay or a similar cream to treat achy pains.

Another way to get almost instant pain relief is through heat. Your options include soaking in a warm bath, wrapping the joint in a warm washcloth, using on-the-go heating patches or a reusable heating pouch. Many experience pain relief until the heat stops. It is best to use heat as a source of relief until your over-the-counter pain pills are able to kick in.

Many natural supplements also claim to add in the relief of arthritis pain and swelling. These supplements are nice, as most are natural and safe. However, they do have their pros and cons. The biggest downside is that most aren't designed for immediate relief. They require, continued use to provide long-lasting relief.

The same is true for exercise. It may be difficult to move your achy joints at first, but continued low-impact exercise like yoga can reduce pain, stiffness, and swelling overtime. Remember that preventing or lessening the risk of pain, discomfort, and swelling is just as important as treating it.

Pain Management and Prevention Methods

In the last chapter, we talked about whether instant relief from arthritis pain and inflammation is possible. In this chapter, we are going to go over some ways you can manage and prevent arthritis pain and inflammation.

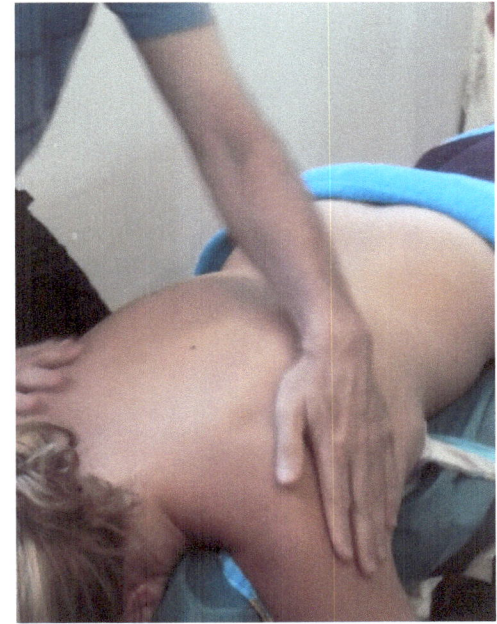

If you suffer from arthritis, pain and inflammation becomes a part of your life. Even those who have dealt with arthritis for years, still suffer. With arthritis, the pain is more than physical. It's emotional too.

When seeking relief, you want more than temporary relief. The best approach is to stop pain before it starts. How? Fortunately, you have many options. Let's go over some of them now:

- Exercise

We coming back to this because exercise is vital to create a strong and healthy body. Not only that, it can relieve and prevent the pain and inflammation associated with arthritis. Those suffering from severe pain, often left their symptoms go untreated.

Their joints are so stiff that it literally hurts to move. If you have reached this point, it will take time. If not, start the process now. Exercise results in joint movement, lessening the stiffness and the pain overtime. It also builds muscle strength. This strength provides the joints with protection, lessening the pressure and pain.

- Protect joints

Those who suffer from severe forms of arthritis suffer every minute of the day. They wake up and feel pain. In fact, a full night's sleep may be near impossible. Prevent joint pain by wisely using your joints and muscles. For instance, if you suffer from arthritis in your elbows or hips? Limit the strenuous activity that requires these joints. Instead of lifting heavy boxes with your arms, lift with the entire body. Instead of turning only the upper part of the body at the hips, reposition the entire body to get a good look.

- Sleep

As I mentioned, sleep can be difficult for those suffering from severe pain. A good night's sleep is vital to preventing pain. The energy the body receives from sleep can ward off pain or lessen its severity. If your nights are restless, sleep whenever possible. This may involve afternoon naps, but the payoff is worth it. A well-rested and well-energized body is able to ward off pain and manage it better.

- Medication in moderation

Unfortunately, those who suffer from pain and inflammation, whether it's arthritis related or not, rely on pain relievers. Some reach the point where they take medication before pain even sets in. They think it will start eventually, so why wait. Don't take this approach, unless advised by a medical professional. The body grows dependent on the medication we ingest. It is easy to become mentally addicted to over-the-counter pain medication. To prevent pain, exercise, eat healthy, and get a good night sleep. Wait until the pain arrives before turning to over-the-counter medication.

- Reduce stress

There is no doubt that arthritis sufferer's deal with pain. However, our bodies play a huge role in the impact it has on our lives. A positive outlook on life will help. The less you focus on your pain, the less you will feel. Relaxation is key too. Does a warm bath relax your body and sooth your joint pain? If so, fill up the bathtub, add scented bubbles, and turn on your favorite music.

- Get a massage

Most patients are surprised to hear their physicians recommend massages. Most assume they will be loaded with pain relievers and sent homes. Yes, over-the-counter relievers do assist with pain, but so does a good old massage. It relaxes the body and mind.

Massages also warm the body and promote movement. In some cases, regular massages can help to prevent pain.

As you can see, there are many ways to avoid and manage the pain associated with arthritis. In fact, these are just a few of your options. No matter what type of arthritis you suffer from or how severe the symptoms, know you are not alone and that relief is available.

Using Food to Control Pain and Inflammation

In the last chapter, we talked about some ways to manage and prevent arthritis pain and inflammation. In this issue, we are going to talk about how some foods that can help relieve arthritis pain and inflammation.

Many who suffer from arthritis use over-the-counter pain medication. In fact, it often becomes a common fixture in their lives. Unfortunately, some individuals are susceptible to addiction and there are health complications due to over-consumption.

If this is the case then it may be time to consider some natural ways to relieve pain and inflammation. You can often start in your kitchen. Although there are no guarantees, many arthritis patients see success by incorporating certain foods into their diets.

What type of foods? Let's go over a few:

- Pineapple

Pineapple is recommended for arthritis because it contains a chemical called Bromelain. Many claims this helps to prevent inflammation. In fact, some athletic trainers recommend its consumption to keep joints pain free and flexible.

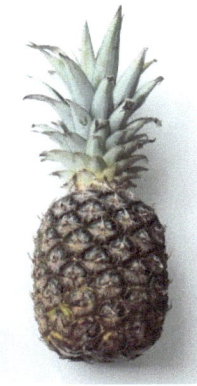

As with any other health foods, it is best to consume fresh instead of canned or frozen.

- Oily fish.

Those suffering from rheumatoid arthritis are often encouraged to avoid meats. Meat has fat that is known to produce inflammation agents in the body. The only exception to this is with fish. Oily fish, such as mackerel and salmon, are rich in omeg-3 fatty acids. These acids have many health benefits. They inhibit the release of joint destroying chemicals and compounds. Supplements are found in most retail stores, but it is best to get these oils directly from the source.

- Celery

The celery plant contains many different anti-inflammatory agents. These can lessen the suffering of arthritis pain and discomfort. It is best to eat the celery seeds. Most recommend placing up to one teaspoon of celery seeds into a cup with warm, but not boiling water. Let stand for a few minutes and drink. This can provide almost instant relief during an attack. The celery plant as a whole contains anti-inflammatory agents; so eating fresh celery regularly has benefits too.

- Red chili pepper.

Red pepper, also known as cayenne pepper, can help relieve the

joint pain associated with 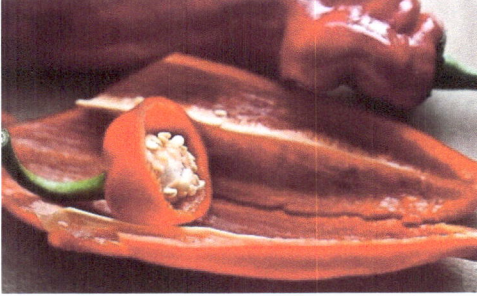 most types of arthritis. As for how, you may be amazed. Many claim it causes the release of natural endorphins. Essentially, your body itself stops the pain. Not only should patients consume red chili pepper, but a topical mixture works too.

Many recommend mixing up to one quart of rubbing alcohol with once ounce of cayenne pepper. It is important to note, this mixture is to be applied to the skin during bouts of pain. Under no circumstances should you drink the mixture due to the rubbing alcohol.

- Sesame seeds

The Chinese have long believed and used sesame seeds to combat the inflammation caused by arthritis. As with oil, sesame seeds contain healthy fatty acids. For the best results, eat sesame seeds straight. If you dislike taste or texture, opt for incorporating them into your meals. Eat sesame seed rolls and use them when preparing dinner at home. They can be added to most foods.

- Ginger

Ginger is well known and widely used to fight inflammation. Most commonly used as a cooking spice, it has many health benefits. In addition to reducing inflammation, it assists in treating diarrhea and nausea. Available in a spice format, it can and should be sprinkled atop cooked vegetables and other foods. As with omeg-3 fatty oils, it is best to go directly to the source. Fresh ginger is easy to peel and cook. Wrapped in a towel, bag, and freeze for months. It is also found in the non-carbonated ginger ale drink.

- Raw cabbage

Although not as well-known and as popular as the above-mentioned foods, many also claim raw cabbage assists with arthritis relief. Some recommend the regular consumption of raw cabbage or cabbage juice. They claim this relieves both joint pain and swelling.

While the foods we discussed in this issue may help reduce the pain and inflammation associated with arthritis, unfortunately, there are no guarantees. Our bodies each process food in different ways.

For instance, celery can work to reduce joint pain for one individual, but it may actually trigger additional pain with another. In fact, some forms of rheumatoid arthritis are trigged by certain foods. For that reason, be prepared to experiment.

Trial and error can help you determine which foods are the best at relieving your own, unique pain and inflammation.

In the book *__101 Superfoods That Stop Joint Pain and Inflammation,__* the author covers several more foods which can work to ease joint pain and inflammation.

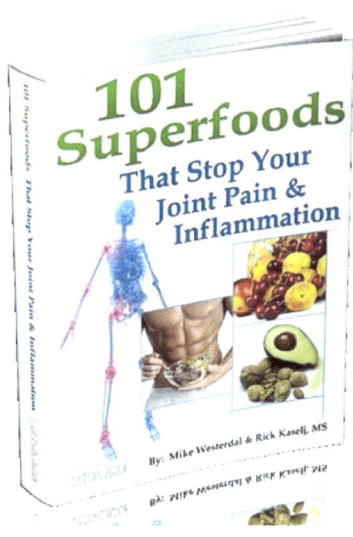

Pain Relief Options While Driving

In the last chapter, we talked about foods that can help relieve arthritis pain and inflammation. In this one, we are going to go over some tips to help ease arthritis pain while driving.

Those suffering from arthritis may find it difficult to walk to the 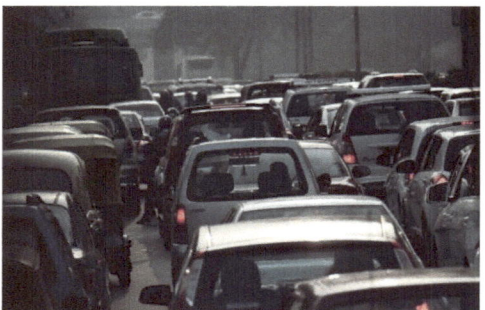 car and back. However, most don't let arthritis stop them from enjoying their life. So, you may head out of the house and hop into your car. This is great, what if you start experiencing pain? How do you treat it on the road or prevent that pain from coming back the next time?

Keep arthritis pain relievers in the car. In one of your car's compartments, have a few pain relief supplies on hand. This may include over-the-counter pain pills, a tube of arthritis cream, or on-the-go heat patches.

Whether you experience pain as soon as you get in your car, or later down the road, rely on these over-the-counter products to seek relief. If you live in an area with cold winters, don't keep these items in your car, as they may freeze. Instead, put them in your purse or briefcase.

Speaking of over-the-counter products, most retail stores sell on-the-go heating patches. These patches stick to your body and warm with skin contact. ThermaCare is a well-known brand. They are ideal when you can't use an electric or microwaveable heating pad. If in pain before you leave the house, but must still leave, like for a holiday party or a doctor's appointment, apply an on-the-go heated patch. Relief will last for up to 12 hours. Since they stick directly to the skin, no adjustments should be needed.

Buy a remote car starter. If you live in the northern United States, it is important to warm your car first. Unfortunately, this may mean an extra trip back and forth. It doesn't have to. Instead, purchase a remote car starter. This device allows you to start and warm your car from inside your home. They also make it easier to unlock car doors. Instead of fumbling with the keys, push the button and your car doors unlock! When buying a remote car starter, look for stores that offer free or discounted installation.

Buy no slip steeling wheel covers. Those who suffer from arthritis of the fingers, dread driving. In fact, some may fear the danger they put themselves and others in. If you find it difficult to grip your car's steering wheel, make a new purchase. That purchase should be an easy grip and no-slip steering wheel cover. Ask a store employee, family member, or friend to install the cover for you.

Keep a jar opener in the car. If you have arthritis of the hands, you likely already utilize rubber jar openers at home. They make griping, twisting, and turning easier. Keep one in your car. Use it to unscrew your car's gas cap. You can also find arthritis gas cap wrenches available for sale. They slip over your gas cap, have an extended and easy grip handle. These are nice, but they can be hard to find. For the same price, you could easily buy 20 rubber jar openers, which accomplish the same goal.

Keep your car well gassed. As I mentioned, there are tools available to make opening and losing the gas cap easier. Even with these tools, it can still be difficult and painful. To prevent the onset of pain, always have a full tank of gas in your car. You won't be forced to put gas in when you are already in pain or more susceptible to it. If you have a full-service gas station in your area, use it.

There are many things that can be done to ease pain while in the car. Just because you suffer from arthritis and are prone to pain, it does not mean you need to live your life in fear. Implement the above-mentioned steps to reduce pain. When it does arrive, turn to your stash of over-the-counter arthritis care products to seek relief.

Treating Rheumatoid Arthritis Early

When diagnosed with rheumatoid arthritis, many patients instinctively prepare for a life filled with pain. Yes, this may be true in some cases. However, a growing number of rheumatologists now believe that this form of arthritis can literally be stopped in its tracks. According to the popular

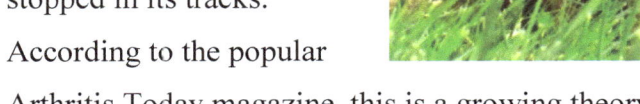

Arthritis Today magazine, this is a growing theory. So, what does it mean for you?

If you suspect you are suffering from arthritis, it is important to seek immediate medical care. Common symptoms of rheumatoid arthritis include joint pain, inflammation, swelling, stiffness, trouble sleeping, and decreased mobility. Treatment options do vary, but a proper diagnosis is key.

There are over one hundred different types of arthritis. Although the treatments are similar, a diagnosis is important. Start with your primary care physician. He or she may later suggest you visit an arthritis specialist, also commonly known as a rheumatologist.

Treatment options for rheumatoid arthritis typically include over-the-counter pain medication. This is to lessen the severity of the pain. Unfortunately, this relief is short lived. That is why many prescribe medication.

When taken overtime, these medications work to combat arthritis. As for the importance of early treatment, the ***Arthritis Today*** magazine highlighted a study performed on the drug Humira. It showed that those diagnosed early were more likely to enter into remission in as little as two years!

Another important aspect of treatment is exercise. Excessive use of the troublesome joints can trigger pain. For that reason, patients need to start slow. For instance, a patient suffering from arthritis of the fingers should move and stretch their fingers daily.

Low impact exercises can relieve joint stiffness and lessen the likelihood of deformities. While pain is likely to increase at first, the more a joint is safely used, the more relief and freedom of movement you are likely to see.

In addition to exercise, healthy eating is important. Combined, the two should result in weight loss. Not all arthritis sufferers are overweight, but some are. This increases pain, as the extra body weight applies more pressure to joints.

With some patients, the pain is trigged by certain foods. Most see success by eliminating or reducing meat and dairy intake. In terms of natural remedies, nothing is scientifically proven, but as we discussed in a previous issue many patients report relief after consuming pineapples, cayenne pepper, raw cabbage, and cold-water fish.

As for why early treatment is important, it slows the progression of the disease. Juveniles are the only individuals likely to outgrow rheumatoid arthritis. For adults, the disease will only progress and get worse, especially without treatment. The health complications are far too great to not do everything you can to help prevent progression and health complications that may lead to severe limitations, disability, loss of mobility, and even deformities.

Legal Notice

The Publisher has strived to be as accurate and complete as possible in the creation of this book, notwithstanding the fact that he does not warrant or represent at any time that the contents within are accurate due to the rapidly changing nature of the Internet.

The Publisher will not be responsible for any losses or damages of any kind incurred by the reader whether directly or indirectly arising from the use of the information found in this publication.

This book is not intended for use as a source of legal, business, accounting or financial advice. All readers are advised to seek services of competent professionals in legal, business, accounting, and finance field.

No guarantees of income are made. Reader assumes responsibility for use of information contained herein. The author reserves the right to make changes without notice. The Publisher assumes no responsibility or liability whatsoever on the behalf of the reader of this book.

This book may contain affiliate programs and advertisements for monetization, which can result in commissions or advertising fees being earned for purchases made by visitors that click through any of the advertisements and/or links included in this text.

About the Author

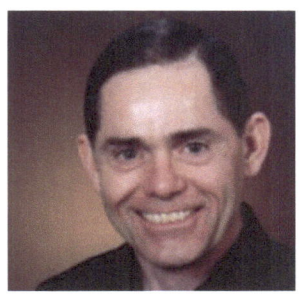

I grew up in Central Minnesota, where my parents own and operated a fishing resort. Once out of high school I tried a couple of semesters of college, only to quit halfway through the Spring term; I decided at that time that college wasn't for me.

Then I decided to follow my father's previous occupation as an auto mechanic. I graduated from a two-year of vocational training course and worked as a mechanic. While in vocational training, I decided to join the National Guard where I eventually ended up working full-time for 32 years.

So how does all of this relate to writing? In one of my leadership schools, the instructor, who was an English teacher at a juvenile detention center, presented writing to me in a whole new way - a way that started to develop my interest in working with words.

Fast forward about 40 years and I now have over 20 books listed on Amazon for Kindle. All of my books with the exception of one children's book (One, Two, Three, Four . . . Counting is Fun at the Grocery Store) are non-fiction in various fields, such as:

*Health and Fitness:

- What You Eat Can Hurt You

- Eat Healthy to Lose Weight

- The Extreme Weight Loss Plan

- Get Ripped Abs

- Walking Down the Road to Fitness

- Design Your Ultimate Fitness Program - Walking

- A Healthier You in the Coming Year

- Senior Fitness – A Guide to Staying Young Beyond Your Years

- Managing Type 2 Diabetes Using Alternative And Natural Therapies

- How Diet and Exercise Can Better Manage Type 2 Diabetes

* Self-Publishing:

- Writing for the Kindle

- How to Self-Publish Your Ebook on Amazon

- Pillars of Gold

- The Beginner's Guide to Fly Tying

- Hooked on Fly Fishing

- The Secrets to Fly Fishing for Trout

- Tent Camping – The Ultimate in Family Fun

- Maintaining a Salt Water Pool

* Misc.:

- Making Wine from Kits

- Create Your Home Inventory

- The 9 Secrets to Using Your GI Bill Benefits

- The Life and Times of the Honey Bee

- The Military Spouses Financial Guide to Funding Education

- The Home-Based Entrepreneur's Guide to Blogging

Survival Basics – Are You Prepared to Survive?

Besides my own writing, I also ghostwrite ebooks, reports, articles, blogs and do Kindle conversions for my clients.

Oh . . . did I mention that I went back to college in 1987 and graduated 7 years later?

Today my wife and I live in Gold Canyon, AZ, where you'll find me happily sitting in my office typing away on my laptop as I work on my next book or ghostwriting project . . . that is if we are not traveling on a cruise ship - our new-found mode of travel.

If you like my book, please leave a review of it on Amazon at the book link above.

www.ingramcontent.com/pod-product-compliance
Lightning Source LLC
Chambersburg PA
CBHW050826290526
45792CB00001B/275